THE COMPLETE KETO DIET FOR BEGINNERS 2022

THE PERFECT MIND IN HEALTHY BODY

Imad Sayli

THE COMPLETE KETO DIET FOR BEGINNERS 2022

TABLE OF CONTENTS

Submit

Many people have different emotions about whether the Ketogenic diet is good for you or not; as someone who follows the Ketogenic diet, I will explain why I believe it is extremely beneficial to your health. It's obviously not for everyone right now, but if it's something you've been thinking about lately, let me help you relax.

The ketogenic diet is a highly effective weight-loss plan. It burns fat rather than glucose since it has a high fat content and a low carbohydrate content. Many people are familiar with the Atkins diet, but the ketogenic diet restricts carbohydrates even more. Avoiding carbohydrates can be difficult when we are surrounded by quick foods and refined foods; but, preparation can help. Here are a few of the keto diet's items.

As more people adopt the "ketogenic diet," more people are beginning to wonder if this is the right diet for them. Even if you're not following a ketogenic diet, you'd be hard-pressed to find such goods in your local supermarket right now. Sellers are aware that the ketogenic diet isn't going precisely where they want it to go, so they begin to prepare tasty "ready-to-go" snacks. Could you please help me?

CHAPTER ONE: DIET THAT IS HEALTHY:

1.What is a Diet Meal Plan for a Healthy Diet?

Knowing what foods to avoid and what foods to eat can help prevent and cure gout, a kind of arthritis caused by an unusually high quantity of uric acid in the blood. Urika is a chemical that emerges as your body breaks down purines, a natural substance found in all cells of your body and the food you eat.

Dark fruit is one of the healthy and delicious foods to eat if you have gouty arthritis.

What exactly are these? What exactly are these? Cherries, blackberries, blueberries, and violet grapes are all good choices. Cherry consumption has been linked to decreased levels of uric acid in recent research. Cherries can be substituted for such items in a variety of dishes. You could prepare cherry pancakes instead of banana pancakes, for example. Consult your doctor to find out which fruits can help supplement your gout diet, as well as which diets are appropriate for you.

In everyday situations, people assume that health is a living being who is free of illness, and it is also difficult to define what health is, but health may be sustained by excellent habits and a well-balanced diet. The key to excellent health is the adoption of healthy eating habits. We've attempted to define a balanced diet meal plan below, using recommendations and tips, so you can handle it according to your needs and desires.

1. The first stage in a well-balanced diet is to divide your daily meal into five or six smaller portions, with each meal lasting one or two days.

2. If you're hungry, include healthful and appetizing meal snacks.

3. Make a one-week meal plan, with a variety of meals and ingredients on hand. Snacks must be prepared ahead of time.

4. Cut off fast food, candies, ice cream, cookies, and chocolates from your diet.

5. You can include crackers, dried and fresh fruit, popcorn, milk, pretzels, low-fat cheese, baby carrots, popcorn air, peanut butter, and almonds and seeds in your diet.

6. Drink more water throughout the day, especially before meals. It keeps your body hydrated and makes you feel less hungry.

7. Cut back on fats and discourage the use of a lot of milk, margarine or butter, poultry, or mayonnaise, and cook with less oil.

8. Vitamin levels in soft drinks and juices are increased to prevent them from being consumed.

9. Include additional grains in your diet by substituting whole grain bread for white bread and brown rice for brown rice.

10. Eat veggies at every meal and avoid high-frequency sugar items.

11. Never skip breakfast because your metabolism increases and your appetite diminishes as the day progresses.

12. Feed gently, and don't give them much more to eat. Because eating is frequently uncontrolled when studying or watching television.

13. Count how many of each dish you have so that you can utilize them in the preparation of a dietary meal plan.

14. When you cook fundamental foods, you can consume a wide variety of foods and eat practically every healthful thing on a regular basis.

15. You can also pack a lunch consisting of tasty sandwiches. It keeps you away from junk food and fast food, and it even includes a list of sandwiches to change up the taste every now and then.

16. Instead of repeating the same meal on the same day, employ a variety of foods for all meals.

17. Stock your cabinets and refrigerator with wholesome foods. Simple, quick-to-prepare ingredients and tried-and-true recipes will help you stick to your diet plan.

18. A balanced diet meal plan should include two vegetarian meals, two fish meals, one fowl meal, and one red meal every week.

19. Purchase a wide variety of fruits and vegetables and include a variety of veggies in each meal.

20. Make meal plans that include safe cooking methods. There will be no more fried food. There will be no more fried meals.

21. You may also appreciate other favorite foods that have a larger calorie count but are consumed infrequently.

22. You can burn extra calories by combining your food plan with an activity routine.

23. Find out what vitamins, minerals, and calories a food form contains, and then follow the diet meat plan you or your family devised for yourself.

2.When it comes to meal planning, there are a few things to consider.

Carbohydrates (necessary for the body's energy generation), protein (important for managing and sustaining physiological processes and a substantial amount of the macro mass of the body), and fat (cellular structure, immune system function, and hormonal production) are the three basic components of the diet. These can be found in a variety of foods. Our bodies meet and maintain their weight and overall health when we eat new, nutrient-dense foods and balance our diet with nutritious carbohydrates, proteins, and fats. With the foods listed below, you should aim to find the right balance to nourish your body.

These foods, in terms of frequency, quantity, and time of day, are critical to your energy, appearance, and general health. The groups that you can include in your daily diet plan and what they accomplish for your body are described below.

Protein sources - (vegetarian, non-vegetarian)

- Sources of milk
- Fruits and veggies
- Fats
- Fruit
- Carbohydrates
- Starches
- Once a Day

What is the purpose of protein in the body?

Protein is necessary for a healthy body because it aids cell expansion and healing. Protein amino acids are the fundamental building blocks of all cells. Protein is essential in our meals when you consider that the human body is a complex biological organism made up of trillions of cells that die and need to be replaced on a daily basis.

Did you know that your digestive tract is replaced every 28 days or so?

That's correct! That's correct! Every 28 days, the cells in our digestive system are completely replaced.

Protein is also beneficial since it helps to regulate blood sugar levels. Amino acids are also needed to develop lean muscle mass in the body. The molecular structure of proteins is extremely complicated. It also takes more energy for the body to digest protein.

Simply put, protein-rich foods cause you to burn more calories! It's excellent to diversify your protein sources by eating a variety of foods and looking for proteins derived from plants and animals.

* * * Not all proteins are manufactured in the same way. Nuts, entire grains, and vegetables are high in protein. However, they do not include all 9 essential amino acids that your body needs to build lean muscle.

* * * * * Vegetarians must use a little more ingenuity to guarantee that the body's required amino acids are stored. One common blunder is

not consuming complete proteins, which do not include all of the needed amino acids.

Combining incomplete proteins with complementary foods is one way to overcome this difficulty. Peanut butter on whole wheat toast or brown rice beans are two examples. Full proteins can be found in vegetarian sources such as hemp seed, tofu, sweet wheat, and quinoa (which contain all essential amino acids).

Milk dairies:

Dairy is part of a balanced middle plan for a variety of reasons. Dairy can provide calcium, added protein during the day, be used as a condiment, or contain important probiotics (found in yogurt) that are beneficial to digestive health. Weight loss is aided by a healthy digestive system.

* * * Cheese is a dairy product that can also be used as a protein source in a vegetarian diet. It can, however, be quite caloric, and more than a share of the food can be easily consumed. Catch 1 oz is a great way to get some cheese into your diet. Serving cheese with a carbohydrate or veggie.

Fat can help you lose weight and improve your overall health:

Fats are necessary in the body because they aid in the transport and absorption of fat-soluble vitamins. Fats are necessary for our overall health and the protection of our internal organs. Avocados and almonds are excellent for reducing inflammation in the body. Fats, both saturated and unsaturated, are essential. Transfats should be avoided at all costs.

Vegetables are your best friend when it comes to losing weight and keeping it off.

Choose a variety of vegetables to add variety to your meal. Combine the ingredients and prepare them so you can enjoy them. Raw and cooked foods can coexist since they both provide healthful carbohydrates, fiber, and a little amount of protein. Vegetables, in particular, provide the body with vital macronutrients, of which many people are deficient. New vegetables can also help to reduce inflammation in the body.

* Important for vegetarians: Make sure to use the "Veg" type for vegetarians.

* * People with hypothyroidism should avoid consuming raw cruciferous vegetables. Cauliflower, broccoli, Brussels sprouts, asparagus, chocolate, cucumbers, bell peppers, garlic,

turmeric, mustard greens, greens, and turf are all cruciferous vegetables. People with hypothyroidism are also thought to be affected by soy products.

Once Every Day Starch:

The Once Regular Starch category includes any entire grain. Foods in this category are high-energy foods that help the body maintain a healthy nutritional balance and are necessary for energy generation. When striving to lose weight, it is critical to consider serving sizes. Stars play a crucial role in the human body.

Blood glucose and insulin levels are sensitive to excess in the body without these carbohydrates. Consider them to be slow carbs. If you're having trouble losing weight, try putting them in your breakfast to stimulate your body to burn the carbohydrates throughout the day.

Sugar divides all carbs into starches. The fiber in these starches slows down the absorption of sugar. Carbohydrates must be appropriately utilized by your body. The importance of quality cannot be overstated.

Fruit: The fruit is absolutely delicious! Fruits are fantastic! They have a natural sweetness and a high fiber content. They also provide the body with important macronutrients and antioxidants. Fruits are necessary for the healing of cellular damage. Only portion proportions should be known in order to prevent future fruit weight increases.

Herbs: Herbs are most effective when they are fresh and unprocessed. They aid in the reduction of inflammation in the body and can enhance the flavor of meals.

It's all about portion control and food preservation. You don't have to be a perfectionist or a zealot to be successful. All you have to do now is drive towards equilibrium.

3.The Benefits of a Meal Plan Diet.

A food plan diet is a good option for long-term weight loss. There are hundreds of diet regimens to choose from. Some have stood the test of time, while others are just around the corner. If you're like the majority of people, you'll move from one plan to the best one for you. Whether or if you lose weight is determined by the strategy itself.

You won't lose weight no matter what it promises if it's poorly put together. If you find a diet plan that promises to help you lose weight rapidly and easily, run the other way.

Weight loss is a difficult task that demands discipline and commitment. It's even more difficult than losing weight. The most effective diet allows you to lose weight and keep it off.

A diet for a meal plan has numerous advantages:

Assist you in achieving a healthy diet. You select meals from each of the food groups required to prepare each meal when creating meals. When you eat well, your body operates better and learns how to burn fat more efficiently. As your metabolism increases, you burn more calories.

You provide flexibility. Allow for some leeway. You can eat a variety of foods while sticking to the meal plan diet. You should eat foods that would be deemed cheating on other diet regimens, and it just becomes a part of the meal by incorporating other 'wants.' You won't be able to eat any pizza, but you may make the diet much easier to follow by limiting some of your favorite meals.

Help in portion control. Help in portion control. We often know how many calories we want to consume during the day, but we struggle to find the correct nutrient mix. How many calories from fats, carbohydrates, and fiber do we require?

It saves both time and money. By not ordering food in advance and instead preparing your meals, you will save money at the grocery store. You write a list and stick to it. Even if you want something from the balanced menu, you can't eat fast food while cooking your meals.

The majority of meal plan diets encourage eating several small meals throughout the day. This boosts the body's metabolism, allowing it to burn calories more efficiently. Most people require only a few hundred calories per meal to keep healthy and satisfied, and only a few hundred calories to lose weight.

4.Diets - Dealing with Setbacks.

Life is a trial-and-error process in which failure and success are two sides of the same coin.

What makes nutrition different?

Dieting is similar to most other things in some ways and different in others.

Because success and failure are two sides of the same coin, the situation remains the same.

It's different because, let's face it, you don't want to diet in the first place.

You're also likely to experience unfavorable dietary thoughts and feelings.

Everyone wants to go on a walk, read a book, drive a car, have a successful career, and be a good friend. Nobody needs to go on a diet.

"Dieting" has a bad meaning.

Then, if you struggle or fall off your diet, you prefer to exaggerate your insufficiency, finding an excuse – conscious or unconscious – to quit, because you began the diet with negative thoughts and sentiments.

And when you break your diet, you begin to see yourself as a failure, which causes your ego, self-confidence, and self-esteem to plummet.

The grief for the loss fades over time.

That's when you can try out the latest fad diet. According to the most recent statistics, dieticians "test" four new diets per year on average.

Herein lies the true dietary disparity. That is the problem.

Past mistakes do not teach you how to better your diet. You'll approach your next diet in the same way you approached your previous failed diet. And then there's the one after that, and then there's the one after that.

Certainly, you're altering your eating habits. You progress from a low-fat, high-protein, low-carbon diet to a steady, long-term cardiac diet.

However, you do not alter your eating habits.

It's a fascinating phenomenon. You learned to walk by falling down many times, and each time you fell, you learned something new, and the next time you walked, you were a little smarter.

You don't get any better the next time you fail at a diet and get up and try something else. Or the one after that. Or the one after that.

While every failure in life provides valuable feedback for our minds and bodies to learn how to improve and provide us with more resilient mental abilities for the next attempt, it does not appear to work for diet.

Why isn't dieting working for you?

There are a variety of reasons why failing at a diet does not help you learn to eat properly the next time.

You never stop walking, reading, driving, or doing anything else. You will never willingly "remain" these things and, as a result, you will have given yourself the opportunity to be a "failure" of them. You've never blown your pride, self-esteem, or self-assurance before. You were never given the option of fixing them, failing, or leaving, so you had no choice but to learn from your mistakes.

You regard the rest of your life as a means to an end. Dieting is never an end... it's a means to an end... thus it's a completely different experience. You should abandon "this" diet, knowing that another is just around the way. You finish... well, whatever it is for you: to look and feel sleek and sexy; to land that dream job; to reclaim your pride and confidence; to wear a bathing suit or swim trunks without being shocked; to play with your kids without getting stuck; to impress your friend at your high school meeting; to stay healthy for a long time.... Furthermore, if you avoid or struggle with dieting, you should (and do) blame it on the diet. "Oh, that diet isn't working for me, or at least it wasn't working for me." But you can't blame your car if you continually failing the driver's exam.

You've never learned how to eat properly, despite the fact that you can successfully diet by utilizing all of your inherent strengths. You were encouraged to stroll and read, as well as all of the other things we stated. However, no one has ever taught you your specific Dieting Compatibility Stylet, so you end up executing a difficult task (dieting) without the necessary skills, assistance, or information.

In most areas of life, you can utilize any setback as a learning opportunity to help you achieve your goals. Failure teaches you and toughens you up.

However, because dieting is never your goal or end goal—only it's a means to an end—you're never truly inspired to eat.

Dieting is likely to be confused with your genuine goal—this attractive figure, for example—but you know it isn't at any point.

It's simpler to give up your diet than most other things in life, but avoiding a new diet means you'll always suffer the pain of failing without the benefit of learning something new.

You've had another diet failure when you're already looking forward to your attractive body and aren't any more prepared for the next diet than you were for the previous one.

There are scientifically-based dietary approaches that leverage your natural strengths and approach your diet to accentuate those strengths and bend your approach to your diet to use those strengths to your advantage, regardless of which diet you choose.

The first step is to determine what diet style(TM) you'll be using and how you'll be using it.

Though you believe that dieting should be intuitive, and that all the advertisements lead you to believe that this time will be different, your experience, as well as the experiences of the 75 million adults in the United States who are currently on a diet and will continue to struggle to eat it, shows that it is neither easy nor intuitive.

Dieting successfully is a skill that must be mastered and practiced in order to be successful. It isn't a difficult skill to perfect. However, as most of us have discovered time and time again, dieting without a diet is nearly impossible to achieve.

Performance and failure are two sides of the same coin.

It's time to put diets in their proper context, learn from past failures, and apply what we've learned to make the next diet the final diet.

If you do it correctly, you can walk or drive your automobile just as easily.

5.Diets That Aren't Fad.

What's the best way to figure out what works and what's good for so many different diets?

The easiest strategy to ensure you learn about the author's background and the study that led to the nutritional approach is to look into his or her history. Any effective diet should include the author's background and experience in the domains of nutrition and biochemistry. However, a broad overview does not imply a healthy and reliable diet. At the very least, it shows that the author has some dietary knowledge. The study behind the diet demonstrates that the diet was not created by a scientist, as the research does not serve itself and adjusts to a theory.

Some diets don't necessitate a slew of tests and studies since they focus on the fundamentals. Many feminine magazines, for example, feature articles on nutrition and weight loss, but it is reasonable to assume that most people who are concerned about their weight are already aware of classic ideolo- gies such as "eat smaller foods," "reduce sugar and fat," and so on. More organized diets, as well as athletes, should provide scientific explanations for their suggested success, preferably case studies and regular test testing.

Because we've agreed to adopt a balanced diet to choose healthy foods and that RDA minimum should be collected, diets may now be generated using those basic characteristics. Begin with a score of 200 and subtract 10 points for each statement below that grants the diet. A score of 200 is ideal, but a score of 160 or higher is acceptable.

1.A diet that lacks sufficient amounts of several food groups. Some outdated diets eliminate one or more food groups. When the nutrients of one food category (e.g., calories, proteins, fats, fibers, vitamins, and minerals) are correctly supplied by those of another food group, do not deduct 10 points.

2.The diet does not get at least 45 percent of its calories from carbohydrate sources. To avoid ketosis, you'll need at least 150 grams of glucose every day. That's 33-50 percent of the total calories consumed in 1200 calories. Take into consideration that this is the bare minimum. This number can rise to 60% for particularly active persons at times, such as shortly after exercise.

3.The carbohydrate quality is more than 20% concentrated sugar. Ideally, at least 80% of the carbohydrate source should come from complex carbohydrates such as fruits, seeds, and legumes.

4.The protein content is greater than 30%. Protein is harmful, puts additional strain on the urinary system, and is a low-energy source. Also, 30 percent is more than plenty for growing youngsters and teenagers. Only people who have recently had serious injuries (e.g., leg amputation), illnesses, or surgeries require increased protein doses. These folks, on the other hand, are treated by a doctor with a high-protein diet.

5.Protein accounts for no more than 15% of total calories. Protein serves numerous critical tasks, including tissue re- pair and enzyme creation, even when consumed in enormous quantities.

6.Fats account for more than 30% of total consumption. High-fiber diets have not been proved to reduce weight better than other 'correct' eating practices, in addition to increasing the risk of cardiovascular disease.

7.The net amount of fat consumed is less than 15% of total calories. Fat, in moderation, is essential for a well-balanced diet and provides many foods flavor.

Fat intakes of less than 15% over lengthy periods of time are impractical for most people. A low-fat diet can harm children and teenagers, who require a lot of calories to grow properly.

8.The total fat intake is less than 25% necessary fatty acids, and saturated fat accounts for more than 30% of total fat consumption. Ten points are deducted for each of them.

9.The diet excludes traditional foods, implying that items can be acquired at any grocery store or market.

10.Dietary foods are either expensive or boring. Many diets stipulate that meals or expensive "organic" items be purchased exclusively from health food stores. Some dishes have such a horrible taste that it's difficult to eat them again and again (e.g., seaweed). Ten points are deducted for each of them.

11.The diet consists of an inflexible meal plan. The diet forbids substitutions or variations, allowing a person to live a 'home-ar- rested' lifestyle with the same meal options every day.

12.The diet contains less than 1200 calories per day. More than that, and your body's essential systems may not receive the energy, vitamins, and minerals they require to function properly, and your dietitian will virtually constantly be hungry. Diets under 1200 calories should be reserved for people under the supervision of a dietician or professional physician.

13.There is a need to augment the food. Supplements are not required if the diet is energy-saving and well-balanced. Weight reduction can be accelerated with 'fat accelerators,' such as ephedrine, but the diet must be able to maintain itself. Some food clinics promote a wide range of fat accelerators and herbal preparations, and these clinics are in business to make money, not as nutritionists.

14.The diet does not specify a realistic weight loss goal. Diets aren't designed to promote the physique of a Greek god or a supermodel. You should not advise someone to drop 100 pounds (even if overweight is 100 pounds).

Diets do not recommend losing weight below your ideal weight.

15.The diet recommends or stimulates a weekly weight loss of more than 1-2 pounds. You ought to Expect to shed no more than 1-2 pounds of fat per week unless you are persistently obese; in this case, 3 pounds may be attainable. A loss of water and/or muscle tissue causes the body to change if more than two pounds are lost every week. Gimmicks that promise you'll lose 10 pounds in two weeks are either not true or promise you'll lose anything other than fat. Remember that the more weight a person has to lose and the less weight they have, the tougher and slower it will be to drop more weight.

16.There is no way to measure dietary habits with this diet. Diet should be a gradual process in which a person's eating habits are altered. It excludes the pursuit of quick fixes and techniques that promise quick fixes or significant changes — no one will ever stick to these programs, and those diets do not work long-term. The number of calories ingested, the dietary variety, and the amount consumed should all be reevaluated on a regular basis... Perhaps once every 1-2 months to analyze the program's success.

17.As part of a weight-loss approach, regular exercise is not recommended.

With exercise, weight reduction occurs twice as quickly, and there is a greater risk of losing lean muscle tissue and fat without it. That's not acceptable.

OVERVIEW OF MANY DIETARY OPTIONS

Low-carbohydrate diets: ketosis is a state of ketosis that has the same drawbacks as fasting. After glycogen is depleted (which occurs frequently in athletes), glucose should be created from protein sources, which is less taxing on the kidneys. Even with a high-protein diet, some protein is withdrawn from body tissue to ensure that the nervous system has enough energy to keep up with everyday exercise. Regardless of what fatty authorities say, the onset of ketosis is a symptom that this phase has begun and is not a desirable aspect.

Because carbohydrates retain water in muscles in a 1:3 ratio, a low carb diet causes significant weight reduction.

Water retention falls when carbon intake decreases. Due to a lack of glycogen, a large amount of water is flushed to retain water molecules. Furthermore, as the youngsters consume water to dilute the nitrogen content, surplus nitrogen flushes with even more water by increasing protein consumption.

Fluid levels rise after leaving a low-carb diet and loading muscles with glycogen, and the dietary supplement regains some weight.

Protein-rich low-calorie diets have the same issues as fasting and low-carbohydrate diets of 400-600 kcals: proteins are utilized to minimize energy, while water is used to extract the majority of the weight. Low-calorie diets should be closely supervised by a physician and used only as a last resort for those who have failed to reduce weight using other methods. Even those people, however, appear to regain a significant amount of weight when they convert to a healthy diet.

The Beverly Hills Diet is a low-mineral, low-vitamin diet consisting of grapefruit, eggs, rice, and celp; minerals and vitamins are in short supply.

The Cambridge diet is a high-calorie (300-600 kcal a day) diet that includes a combination of protein and carbohydrates, as well as mineral imbalances, and the dieter is on the verge of fasting.

"Fake" Mayo diet - consists of grapefruits, eggs, rice, and kelp; deficit in minerals and vitamins.

F-Plan Diet – is a calorically diluted high fiber (30-35g/day) diet; it is low in fat and animal products; mineral absorption is poor due to fiber.

LA Costa Spa Diet – This diet promotes weight reduction of 1-1 pound a day and is divided into three parts: 800, 1000, and 1200 calories per day. It is made up of 25% protein, 30% fat (mostly polyunsaturated), and 45 percent carbohydrate.

The Medifast Diet is nutritionally sound, however it only provides 900 calories a day, making the use of liquid formula monotonous and pricey.

The Nutriment Diet, also known as the Medifast Diet, is a nutritionally balanced diet that provides just 900 calories per day, making it monotonous and expensive due to the use of liquid formulae.

The Optifast diet is nutritionally sound, however it only delivers 900 calories per day. Liquid formulations are tedious and expensive.

The Pritikin Permanent Weight-Loss Diet is nutritionally unbalanced; certain days have calorific constraints; the diet moves quantities of carbohydrate, protein, and fat; the diet is based on high protein (100 g per day); vitamin B12 absorption is limited unless appropriately selected foods are consumed.

Prudent diet-a healthy diet of 2400kcal per day for men, low in cholesterol and saturated fats; fat derived from a maximum of 20-35 percent of calories, with an emphasis on protein, carbohydrates, and salt; adequate intake of fish and shellfish, and polyunsaturated fats are supplemented with saturated fat.

This diet is nutritionally unbalanced; caloric limitations some days; the dieter varies sections of carbohydrate, protein, and fat, while low carbohydrates (20-50 g/day) and high fat and protein are consumed; meat (saturated fat and cholesterol) is consumed with this diet.

The diet begins with 500 calories per day, consisting of two meals a day with one fruit, one potato, one slice of bread, and two exchanges of meat; the second week restricts the amount of carbohydrates, with the majority of foods coming from the meat community, eggs and cheese, and some vegetables; the third week adds fruit; the fourth week increases the number of vegetables; and the fifth week introduces the amount of fat cooked by the dieter;

Slendernov Diet - this diet is nutritionally unbalanced; certain days are low in calories; the dietary diet changes the percentages of carbs, protein, and fat; protein is big in general (100 g / day); vitamin B12 may be inadequate unless the food is correctly picked.

Weight monitor diet – this diet is nutritionally balanced, containing roughly 1000-1200 kcal; a high-nutrient diet is consumed; inexpensive and pleasant food is ingested; this diet is one of the most popular diets with no actual health hazards.

A wine diet—roughly 1200 kcal/day, 28 menus, and a slice of dry table wine for dinner; in addition to the therapeutic components of wine, people are believed to reduce the portion of their diet when eating wine; cholesterol- and saturated fats—low ; fish, poultry, and veal with moderate amounts of red meat are the main components of this diet.

Yogurt Diet — with a daily caloric intake of 900 to 1000 kcal and a daily caloric intake of 1200 to 1500 kcal, yogurt is a high-protein, low-cholesterol, low-saturated-fat, and low-refined-carbohydrate food.

CHAPTER TWO:BEGINNER'S KETO DIET:

6.What exactly is Keto?

Glucose is generally the body's primary source of energy. Your body converts its fuel supply to fat when you eat very few carbs and moderate amounts of protein (extra protein can be converted to carbohydrates). Fatty ketones are produced by the liver (a fatty acid type). These ketones are a source of energy for the body, particularly the brain, which absorbs a lot of it and may run on glucose or ketones.

Ketosis is a metabolic condition that develops when the body produces ketones.

Fasting is the greatest approach to get into ketosis. When you eat a lot of carbs and protein in a short amount of time, your body switches to burning stored fat for heat. As a result, the diet appears to help you lose more weight.

Keto's diet necessitates long periods of eating very little carbohydrate (less than 30 g per day) or nearly no carbohydrate at all, while increasing your fat intake to a high level (to the point where fats make up as little as 65 percent of your total macronutrient intake). The body should be more inclined to utilise fat for energy in this condition of ketosis, according to study. You must finally be shredded once your glucose and glycogen livers are depleted and you switch to fat for fuel.

You follow the specific platform from Monday through Saturday at 12 p.m. (afternoon) (or Saturday at 7 p.m., depending on the version you read). Then, from now until 12 a.m. on Sunday night (up to 36 hours later), drive your huge car...

(Some people believe that you can take nuts into the carbohydrate and eat whatever you like, while others believe that you should only eat clean carbohydrates throughout your carbohydrate, which is also controlled by your body.)

7.The Ketogenic Diet.

For many people, the ketogenic diet is an excellent weight-loss option. It's quite different, and it encourages people to eat a diet that includes foods they can't predict.

As a result, the ketogenic diet, also known as keto, is a low-carbohydrate, high-fat diet. How many times can you start your day with plenty of bacon and eggs, then follow it up with chicken wings for lunch, and then steak and broccoli for breakfast? For others, this may appear to be too good to be true. Yes, this diet is a terrific day to eat, and you followed the meal plan to the letter.

The body enters ketosis when it consumes very few carbs. This means that the body burns fat for energy. How few carbs should you consume in order to enter ketosis? It varies from person to person, but it's best to stay under 25 net carbohydrates. Many experts advise staying under ten net carbs during the "induction" period, which is when your body is bringing itself into ketosis.

If you're not sure what net carbohydrates are, let me assist you. Net carbohydrates are the carbs consumed after excluding dietary fiber. Your net carbohydrate for the day will be 22 if you eat 35 grams of net carbohydrate and 13 grams of dietary fiber. Isn't it simple enough?

And, aside from weight loss, what else does keto have going for it? Many people claim that when on this diet, they have more mental clarity. Another benefit is an increase in energy. Another symptom is a loss of appetite.

When following the ketogenic diet, one thing to keep in mind is the so-called "keto flu." This isn't something that everyone has to deal with, but it can be difficult. You may get fatigue and a headache. It won't last much longer. If you're feeling this way, drink plenty of water and get some rest.

What are you waiting for if this sounds like a diet you'd be interested in?

Dive was first heard in keto. You won't believe what you'll learn in such a short period of time.

8.The Advantages of a Keto Diet

Keto isn't a new way of eating. It began as a medical practice to treat epilepsy in infants in the 1920s, but the diet became blind as anti-epileptic drugs became available. Because of its success in reducing the incidence of seizures in epileptic patients, there is an increasing amount of study being done on the nutritional potential for treating a variety of neurological illnesses and other chronic diseases.

• Diseases of the nervous system. A recent study demonstrates the benefits of keto in the treatment of Parkinson's disease, Alzheimer's disease, autism, and multiple sclerosis. It can also protect the brain from damage and strokes. One theory for keto's neuroprotective properties is that the ketones created during ketosis provide more food to brain cells, which can help them fight inflammatory damage induced by these conditions.

Obesity and weight loss are two topics that come up frequently. If you wish to reduce weight, the Keto diet will assist you in gaining access to and releasing body fat. When it comes to losing weight, the most difficult task is constant starvation. The keto diet helps to prevent this because it improves satiety, which makes it simpler for people to stick to their diets by reducing carbon consumption and boosting fat intake. Obese people who followed a low-carb (20.7 pounds) diet lost twice as much weight in 24 weeks as those who followed a low-fat diet (10.5 lbs).

• Diabetes type 2. The keto diet not only helps people lose weight, but it also improves insulin sensitivity, which is beneficial for people with type 2 diabetes. Diabetics on low-carb keto diets have been able to drastically reduce their diabetes dependence and even reverse it, according to research published in Nutrition & Metabolism. Other health indicators, such as triglyceride reduction and LDL (bad) cholesterol reduction, as well as a rise in HDL (good) cholesterol, are also improved.

• Carcinoma. The majority of individuals are unaware that glucose is the primary source of energy for cancer cells. This indicates that having a healthy diet can assist you from getting cancer. Sugar is the major source of fuel for cancer cells because the keto diet is low in carbohydrates. Healthy cells will use ketones as energy when the organism produces them, but malignant cells will not, as they will starve.

Since 1987, studies on keto diets have demonstrated lower tumor growth and increased survival for a variety of malignancies.

The keto diet differs from regular American and Paleo diets in that it has significantly less carbohydrates and far more fat. Ketones circulating between 0.5 and 5.0 mM are a result of the keto diet. With a home blood ketone detector and ketone test strips, this is possible. (Please keep in mind that urine ketones tests aren't always accurate.)

7 Keto Advantages for Weight Loss

7-Keto-DHEA is a naturally occurring active metabolite of the hormone DHEA that is involved in a variety of bodily activities. 7-Keto-DHEA levels decline over time, but can be returned to normal with supplementation. Basic 7-keto benefits include decreased cortisol, improved immunological function, and faster weight loss and maintenance for users.

How to Put 7-Keto-DHEA to Work

7-Keto-DHEA enhances the pace of weight loss mostly by raising the body's thermogenesis temperature. Other supplements, such as DHEA, caffeine, and ephedrine, boost thermogenesis, but they come with negative side effects including increased blood pressure. One of the most important 7-Keto benefits is improved thermogenesis, which has no negative side effects. Furthermore, 7-Keto can be utilized at extremely high amounts without causing harm. According to one study, test animals were not harmed by taking a 40.000 mg equivalent per day, which is around 200-400 times the average 100 or 200 mg daily prescription dose.

Dieters can benefit from 7-Keto-improved DHEA's metabolic rate even after they've started their diets. Instead of experiencing slowed metabolism as a result of a low-calorie diet, customers experience a stable metabolism and avoid plateau losses.

Thyroid hormone T3 is also increased by 7-Keto. Some weight-loss supplements, such as l-tyrosine, boost fat consumption by increasing T3 levels, although T3 levels always drop when taken. 7-Keto, on the other hand, maintains high T3 levels in users, allowing for sustained weight loss.

Scientists have discovered that this increase in T3 stays within a healthy, natural range, allowing consumers to benefit from increased T3 without experiencing too much decline.

7 Benefits of Keto Diet for Weight Loss

7-Keto-DHEA isn't a weight-loss product that works like magic They can easily lose weight. The major 7 Keto benefits of cortisol reduction, higher T3, and improved thermogenesis, when combined with diet and preparation, make weight loss much easier. The reduction of cortisol, which encourages people to practice more and more during their routines, is one of the seven benefits of Keto. This is only one method that 7-Keto-DHEA can help you lose weight.

7-Keto-DHEA enhances the body's usage of insulin and reduces fat growth, in addition to its other effects. In comparison to other modern weight loss pills, 7-Keto addresses a broader range of issues to give nutritional efforts a significant boost.

9.How To Formulate A Keto Diet?

1.Carbohydrates :

are the primary source of energy.

Most people need to limit their carb intake to 20 to 50 grams (g) per day to achieve ketosis (ketone levels over 0.5 mM). The amount of carbohydrates consumed varies from person to person. In general, the more insulin resistant an organism is, the more ketosis resistant it is. People with type 2 diabetes and insulin resistance may need to eat closer to 20-30 g / day, but insulin-sensitive exercise athletes can eat more than 50 g / day and keep ketosised.

It is permissible to calculate carbs using net carbs, which are total carbs minus fiber and sugar alcohols. The term "net carbon" refers to carbon dioxide, which boosts blood sugar and insulin levels. The fiber has no metabolic or hormonal effect, and neither do most sugar alcoholics. Maltitol is an exception, as it can affect blood sugar and insulin levels without causing major side effects. As a result, if maltitol is listed among the components, sugar alcohol should not be deducted from total carbs.

The quantity of carbon that can be absorbed and kept in ketosis varies over time, depending on keto modifications, weight reduction, workout habits, medicines, and other factors. The ketone levels should subsequently be calculated on a regular basis.

Overall, carbohydrate items such as pasta, cereals, potatoes, rice, beans, candies, sodas, juice, and beer are not well tolerated by most people's diets.

Lactose (milk sugar) carbohydrates are found in almost all milk products. Some, on the other hand, have fewer carbs and can be consumed on a daily basis. Hard cheeses (parmesan, cheddar), mild high-fat cheeses (brie), full-fat milk cheeses, high-fat milk, and sour cream are examples.

A carb intake of fewer than 50 g per day consists of: • 5-10 g of protein-based dietary carbohydrates. Eggs, cheese, and coquillages provide a few extra grams of carbs, as well as natural marinades and spices.

• Vegetables (non-starch): 10-15 g

• 5-10 g carbs from nuts and seeds Per ounce, most nuts contain 5-6 grams of carbohydrates.

Strawberry, olives, tomatoes, and avocados all provide 5-10 g of fruit carbohydrates.

• 5-10 g of carbon from a variety of sources, including low-carb sweets, high-fat dressings, and tiny amounts of sugary beverages.

Beverages

The average person need at least half a gallon of total fluid every day. The best sources include organic coffee, filtered water, tea (unsweetened, regular, and decaf), and non-sweetened amond and cocoon milk. Artificial sweeteners are included in diet drinks and beverages, thus they should be avoided. You should limit your white or red wine consumption to 1-2 glasses per person. If you drink spirits, stay away from sweetened mixed beverages.

2. A source of protein:

A keto diet does not include a lot of protein. This is due to the fact that protein raises insulin levels and can be converted into glucose through a process known as gluconeogenesis, which also avoids ketosis. However, an insufficient protein intake might result in muscle tissue loss and function.

On a daily basis, the average adult gains 0.8-1.5 g of lean body mass per kilogram (kg). It's important to note that the measurement is based on lean body mass rather than total body weight. The reason for this is that fat mass does not require protein, while lean muscle mass does.

If a person weighs 150 lbs (or 150/2.2 = 68.18 kg) and has a body fat content of 20% (or a lean body mass of 80% = 68,18 kg x 0.8 = 54.55 kg), for example, the protein requirement might range from 44 (= 54.55 x 0.8) to 82 (= 54.55 x 1.5) g/d.

People who are insulin-resistant or who are on the keto diet for medical reasons (cancer, epilepsy, etc.) should aim to come closer to the lower protein boundary. The higher limit is for persons who are really healthy or sporty. The daily protein amount for someone else on a keto diet for weight loss or other health advantages should be somewhere between them.

Grass-fed meats (6-9 g protein/oz) and organic eggs (6-8 g protein/egg) are high-quality protein sources, as are animal sources of omega-3 fats including salmon, sardines, and anchovies, and herring, caught in the wild in Alaska. (Protein / 6-9 g / ounce).

• Almonds, macadamia, flax, pecans, sesame seeds, and hemp seeds and nuts (4-8 g protein/4 cup)

• Fruits and vegetables (about 1-2 g protein per ounce)

3. Obesity:

After determining the proper amount of carbohydrates and protein to consume, the majority of the diet is made up of fat. The fat content of a keto diet must be substantial. When adequate fat is consumed, the body's weight is maintained. If weight loss is desired, less calories should be consumed and body fat should be kept for energy expenditure.

Individuals who consume 2000 calories per day consume between 156 and 178 grams of fat per day. Large and highly active adults with high energy demands who maintain their weight can consume up to 300 grams of fat each day.

Most people can handle a high-fat diet, but some conditions, such as gallbladder removal, can limit the amount of fat that can be consumed in a single meal. More regular eating, as well as the usage of bile salts or lipase-rich pancreatic enzymes, may be beneficial.

Stop consuming trans fats, extensively processed polyunsaturated vegetable oils, and large amounts of polyunsaturated omega-6 fats.

The following foods are the best sources of high-quality fats:

• Coconut oil and coconuts

Avocados and avocado oil are two of the healthiest foods you can eat.

• Grass-fed butter, beef fat, and ghee • Organic heavy cream from pastured cows • Olive oil

• Lard from pastured pigs • Medium-chain triglycerides (MCTs)

MCTs are a form of lipid that is digested differently than other long-chain fatty acids. MCTs may be used by the liver to generate energy before glucose, allowing for higher ketones synthesis.

Concentrated sources of MCT oil are available as supplements. Many people use them to help them get into ketosis. The only food that contains MCTs is coconut oil.

MCT accounts up about two-thirds of the cocoa fat.

Who Should Be Wary Of A Keto Diet?

For the most part, a ketogenic diet is really healthful. However, some people should take extra measures and consult with their doctors before beginning such a regimen.

• People who use diabetes medications. As blood sugar levels fall as a result of a low-carb diet, dosage may need to be adjusted.

• People who take blood pressure medications. Because a low-carbon diet reduces blood pressure, the dosage will need to be adjusted.

• Breastfeeding mothers don't need to follow the strictest low-carb diet because their bodies shed roughly 30 grams of carbs per day through milk.

Get at least 50 g of carbs every day while breastfeeding.

• Patients with kidney illness should seek medical advice before embarking on a ketogenic diet.

Typical Keto Diet Concerns

• I couldn't get into ketosis. Make sure you're not eating too much protein and that your meals don't contain any hidden carbs.

- Consume high-processed polyunsaturated maize and soybean oils as a source of fat.
- Symptoms of "keto flu," such as lightheadedness, dizziness, headaches, fatigue, brain fog, and constipation. When in ketosis, the body appears to excrete more sodium. Keto-flu symptoms can develop if you don't obtain enough salt in your diet. This can be easily addressed by drinking 2 cups of broth per day (with extra salt). You may need to add more sodium if you exercise vigorously or have a high perspiration rate.
- The influence of dawn. Unless they are diabetic, standard blood fasting sugars are fewer than 100 mg/dl, and most ketosis patients exceed this amount. When following a keto diet, however, some people's blood sugar levels spike, especially in the morning. Because of the normal circadian surge in morning cortisol (stress hormone), which leads the liver to create more glucose, this is known as the "dawn effect." If this happens, avoid eating too much protein at dinner and sleeping too close together. Cortisol levels can also be influenced by stress and insufficient sleep. If you're insulin resistant, it may take longer to get into ketosis.

• Poor athletic performance. Keto adaption takes roughly four weeks on average.

Instead of intensive exercises or preparation, we switch to something less strenuous at this time. Sports performance usually returns to normal or improves after the adjustment phase, especially in endurance competitions.

• Keto-rash isn't your normal dietary complication. Acetone synthesis in perspiration, comprising protein or minerals, which irritates the skin, and dietary shortages are two possible causes. After exercising, take a shower and make sure all of your foods are thick and nutrient-dense.

• Ketoacidosis is a condition in which the body produces ketones. When blood ketone levels exceed 15 mm, this is an extremely rare occurrence. A well-designed keto diet does not produce ketoacidosis. For SGLT-2 inhibitors, such situations as type 1 diabetes or breast-feeding necessitate extra attention. Vomiting, nausea, tiredness, and shortness of breath are some of the symptoms. Mild instances can be solved with sodium bicarbonate mixed with apple juice or diluted orange. Significant symptoms necessitate immediate medical attention.

Is Keto Safe To Consume For A Long Time?

This is a hotly debated topic. While no studies have shown that a keto diet has any long-term negative consequences, many experts now agree that the body will build "resistance" to ketosis if it is not frequently entered and exited. Furthermore, a high-fat diet for a lengthy period of time may not be suitable for many species.

Cyclical ketogenic diet

It's time to add carbs back into your diet whenever you can consistently produce more than 0.5 mM of ketones in your blood. On those Carb Food Days, instead of eating 20-50 g of carbs each day, you may want to increase it to 100-150 g.

Usually, 2-3 times each week is plenty. It's best if you can do it on days when you're training and eating a lot of protein.

Some folks who are hesitant to replace some of their favorite foods permanently will find this cycle strategy more tempting. It may also make it harder for sensitive people to stick to the keto diet or create binges.

10.Beginner's Guide to the Keto Diet.

Everyone seems to be talking about the ketogenic diet these days: a low-carbohydrate, moderate-protein, high-fat diet that transforms the body into a fat-burning powerhouse. The benefits of this diet have been widely promoted by Hollywood celebs and athletes, ranging from weight loss to preventing inflammation, lowering blood sugar, lowering cancer risk, enhancing energy, and slowing aging. Is keto, however, something you should think about? This will highlight what this diet is all about, as well as the advantages and disadvantages, as well as the concerns.

11.Keto Dieting? Here Are 10 Foods You Must Have in Your Kitchen.

The ketogenic diet is a popular weight-loss plan. It burns fat rather than glucose since it is high in fat and low in carbohydrates. Many people are familiar with the Atkins diet, but the keto technique reduces carbohydrates even further.

Avoiding high-carbon foods can be difficult because we are surrounded by fast-food restaurants and processed foods, but proper preparation can assist.

Plan your dinners and snacks at least a week ahead of time so you don't get caught up in high-quality meals. Look up keto recipes online; there are a lot of good ones to select from. Find and stick to your favorite keto recipes once you've started the keto diet.

A keto diet necessitates the use of certain goods. Check to see if these items are available:

1. Eggs—omelets, hard-boiled eggplant, quiches, low-carb pizza crust, and more may all be made with eggs.

2. Bacon-Do I need a justification for this? Breakfast, salad, burger toppings, and black-berry

ice cream (no toast, of course; try a BLT in a cup, thrown into mayo)

3. Cream cheese—hundreds of meals, pizza crusts, main courses, and desserts

4. cheese that has been shredded in a bowl formed of microwave tortilla chips, salad toppers, low-carb pizza, and shrimp, sprinkle with taco meat.

5. A lot of Romaine and Spinach—Fill the green veggies to make a quick salad when hunger strikes.

6. EZ-Sweetz liquid sweetener – Instead of sugar, use a few drops of this natural and simple-to-use artificial sweetener.

7. Cauliflower-This low-carb vegetable can be eaten alone in fresh or frozen packets, tossed in olive oil and fried, mashed into flaky potatoes, shredded and used as a rice substitute in major dishes, topped with low-carb and keto pizzas, and many other ways.

8. Frozen chicken tenders – Keep a large bag on hand; thaw and barbeque, sauté, combine with vegetables and top with low-carbohydrate garlic

sauce; use in chicken alfedo, chicken piccata, tacos, indigenous butter chicken, and more.

9. Ground beef – Make a large burger with a variety of toppings, such as cheese, sauteed mushrooms, grilled onions... or crumble and cook taco or taco shells with lettuce, avocado, and cheese, as well as sour taco cream for a tortilla taco salad.

10. Almonds (flavored or unflavored)-these are tasty and nutritious snacks, but please keep them in your hands while you eat to avoid accumulating carbs. The flavors include habanero, cocoon, salt and vinegar, and others.

The keto diet is a versatile and exciting strategy to lose weight that offers a variety of delicious meal selections. You'll be able to add some wonderful delicacies and snacks to the fridge, freezer, and pantry in the morning.

A ketogenic diet is a better option for everyone who wants to lose weight. Visit Balanced Keto, a great website that provides dieters with dietary ideas and nutritional facts.

12.Net Carbohydrates.

Carbohydrates that the body can digest and process as dietary carbohydrate are known as net carbs. As a result, blood sugar levels are influenced directly. By subtracting the nutrition, glycerin, and sugar alcohol grams from the total carbohydrate, you may calculate how many net carbs you consume. For low-carb regimens like the Atkins diet, net carbohydrates are the only carbs you can eat.

It's critical to understand why fibers aren't the same as regular carbohydrates. Because fiber does not break down into sugar, it does not contribute to the overall sugar load of the carbohydrate. When a bread slice contains 27 grams of carbohydrate and 3 grams of fiber, the carbohydrate content is just 24 grams (27 g – 3 g = 24 grams).

This explains why certain high-fibre diets have a positive impact on blood sugar and insulin levels.

Dietary fiber is only found in herbal foods. Fiber has a number of advantages as well as some disadvantages when it comes to digestion. Fiber has a number of advantages, including the ability to slow down the digestion of food. As a result, food from the stomach is gradually emptied into the small intestine. This guarantees that large amounts of glucose can be easily taken into the bloodstream from the small intestine, reducing the risk of an insulin shortage. Insulin is a hormone that is secreted from the small intestine when glucose is consumed. Slowing the stomach's emptying may help prevent the body from producing excessive levels of insulin as a result of frequent quick glucose releases into the intestine. In fact, this will aid in the prevention of diabetes in those who are prone to it.

Fiber, on the other hand, is impeded by the absorption of some nutrients. In a moderately heavy fiber diet, this incursion can prevent up to 5% of fat from being absorbed.

This is also good news in Australia, where 63 percent of men and 47 percent of women were overweight in 1995, with no signs of the rate of overweight and obesity declining.

The absorption of a number of vital minerals or trace elements is typically hampered by a high fiber diet, but because a high fiber diet often provides extra minerals and trace elements, the effect is not regarded to be especially important in regular western diets.

Despite these minor side effects, a high fiber intake has been found to be consistently helpful. Low fiber intake, particularly insoluble fibers like those found in bread and other wheat products, is one of the leading causes of constipation. Low fiber intake has also been linked to a higher risk of diverticulitis. In addition to rectal cancer, hemorrhoids, obesity, appendicitis, and colitis ulcers, a lack of fiber in the diet can cause rectal cancer, hemorrhoids, obesity, appendicitis, and colitis ulcers. Reduced blood cholesterol is linked to a high intake of fruits, vegetables, rolling oats, saponins found in legumes, and insoluble fibers like pectin and gum. High consumption of herbal foods, all of which contain some fiber, is linked to a lower risk of cardiovascular disease, cancer, and a longer life expectancy.

Another benefit, and one that can help with weight management, is the feeling of satiety, or a sense of fullness that comes with a high-fiber meal. It's also true that high-fiber meals are generally often low in fat, therefore a high-fiber diet is usually low in fat.

Carbohydrates stored in the body's systems as dietary carbohydrates are referred to as net carbs. Net carbohydrates have a direct impact on blood sugar levels. To calculate your consumption, divide the number of grams of carbs by the number of grams of fiber, glycerine, and sugar alcohol. The net carbohydrate remains the same. This is how much you should use for things like the Atkin diet. It's important to understand that fiber is not a carbohydrate. Fiber does not convert to sugar in your system, thus it does not act as a sugar burden in your body. For example, if a loaf of bread has 27 grams of carbs and 3 grams of fiber, the net carbide content is 24 grams. Gram for gram, the fiber wipes out the fat.

High-fiber diets can raise blood sugar levels. Plants are the only source of dietary fiber. Many fiber benefits have an impact on the digestive system. It delays the absorption of food, ensuring that you obtain more nutrients from your food and avoiding blood sugar or insulin rises. Insulin is a hormone produced by your small intestines in response to the absorption of glucose. By slowing down digestion, fiber can help you avoid creating too much insulin. This will aid the body in consuming the proper nutrients and prevent diabetes in many people.

A high-fiber diet, for example, can flush out around 5% of the fat you consume. The few minerals prevented by fiber will not have an unfavorable effect on a typical Westerner's regular diet because the delayed digestion will absorb several more minerals and vitamins. A high-fiber diet is almost always preferable. Constipation is caused by a lack of fiber in many diets, which can be a major source of discomfort. Rectal and hemorrhoid cancer, appendicitis, ulcerative colitis, and diverticulitis are all caused by it.

13.Menu Options for Low-Carb and Keto Diet Fast Food: How to Eat Successfully at Restaurants.

There is always something to eat for individuals on low carb or keto diets in any fast food or restaurant. Make preparations ahead of time. Before going to a restaurant, look up their menu and nutritional information online or on your phone. It is always important to be aware of healthier alternatives before succumbing to carbohydrate eating temptations.

To make it easier to discover a quick-keto-friendly option, I've produced a list of numerous eateries and fast-food establishments that I consider to be the cheapest (and most emotionally rewarding). They aren't all perfect choices, but if you don't have a choice due to time or location constraints, you make do.

Quick-service restaurants are a big help in delaying the nutritional content. It gets easier to stick to the keto diet every day. The carbohydrate count I offer is an estimate in NET grams.

Almost wherever you go, there is a salad option. At Burger King, the bun is removed, and salad wraps are available at many locations. Breading isn't necessary for chicken.

Breading.

It's also a good idea to keep a knife in your car or wallet. Tall, juicy burgers end up on the table or on the lap in tiny salad pieces. Fast-food plasticware is also difficult to eat since it is so little and flimsy. Remove your utensils and enjoy them!

Now it's time to think about meal options... Here are a few recommendations to follow that are typically self-evident:

• Forego the wrap or bun; forego the potato, rice, or pasta; and forego the croutons in salads. Low-sugar dressing options include ranch, blue cheese, Caesar, and chipotle. Look for names that offer you a hint, such as "honey" in the sweet dressing or "sweet" in the name; these aren't usually smart choices. Look for items having a greater carbohydrate content in the ingredient list.

• Choose between grilled or dusted chicken. Any breaded chicken should be avoided.

McDonald's—choose either grilled chicken (2 g) or (zero-g) burger with no bun and mayo, mustard, onions, and other toppings. There will be no ketchup. There will be no ketchup. Attach the lettuce to the side (3 g). The grilled chicken Caesar salad or the grilled chicken bacon salad are both 9 g.

Burger King: Burger (null g) on a bun with mayonnaise, cheese, onions, and mustard... McDonald's provides the same burger information. There will be no ketchup. There will be no ketchup. The tender grill chicken sandwich weighs 3 g without the bun. BEWARE — the veggie burger may appear little, but it has 19 grams of carbs, which means you'll be eating keto carbs for the rest of the day. BEWARE. Attach the lettuce on the side (3 g). Without dressing or croutons, the garden salad with tender grill weighs 8 g. It's not possible to eat the chicken salad. Don't even attempt. Don't even attempt.

BONUS—a freshly fried apple with 5 g of net carbs and caramel sauce that isn't fried.

If you're lucky, you'll be able to miss Subway-Subway. Carbohydrates abound in the buns and wraps. I suppose you could just put the components in a wrapper without the bread, but that doesn't sound appealing. I don't know how many carbs any single bunless sub would have had, but you can probably figure it out-chicken or pepperoni are good, but "sweet onion" chicken is okay? I have no idea.

I have no idea. Stick to salads and just buy iceberg lettuce (4 g).

Carl's Junior and Hardees-This fast-food business offers a "lettuce wrap," which is a huge piece of lettuce wrapped in lettuce for a quick low-carb meal. I prefer to eat with my own fork.) a six-dollar burger (7 g), a half-pound burger (5 g), and a charcoal chicken club sandwich (7 g/10 g in Hardees). Unless There Are No Alternatives. Grilled chicken salad is 10 g without croutons. On the side, there is a 3 g salad.

In this case, the unwich, a Jimmy John's sandwich wrapped in salad, fits the bill. Food is fine, as long as the ingredients don't have a lot of emissions.

Wendy's is a fast food restaurant chain. You can bring your burger in a lettuce wrap or a packaging once again. Any burger with any toppings. Mayonnaise contains maize syrup and weighs 1 gram. The chicken grill fillet weighs 1 gram. It's available as a chicken sandwich or a chick- en grill ultimate sandwich. Best salads: grilled chicken salad (7 g), chicken caesar (7 g). 6 g or 2 g side salads for Caesar.

Pizza Hut and other pizza-related establishments-

It is possible to eat pizza without the crust. If you can't stop a party or supper at the pizza, just peel off a cheesy top and devour the enormous sloppy mass of cheese and toppings. A side salad is a nice addition. Otherwise, I simply prefer to bake pizza at home with low-carbon crusts.

YES! Mongolian Grill! Fill the bowl with chicken, shrimp, onion, and mushrooms, then pour in the Asian black bean sauce. Although I am aware that beans include carbohydrates, this label specifies 1 gram of carbohydrates per unit (every sauce is a label).

Place a small amount of garlic on top and wait for the griller to finish his work. Appetizers, tortillas, and rice are clearly missing from your menu. Request that the waiting staff not carry them to the table.

Italian restaurants require a bit of foresight, but they can be aggravating!

Consider the Italian chicken Marsala as an example. Make that the pasta does not enter the room. Replace broccoli with a large salad or another keto-friendly side dish. Piccata de chicken is another option.

Mexican and Chinese restaurants are the most difficult because a low carb option is not the primary reason for visiting to the restaurant. In a Mexican restaurant, I like to order a large burrito with no boobs and spread the soft tortilla out like a platform. Eat the inner ingredients and toss the tortilla.

If you absolutely must go to the Chinese buffet (I once attended a funeral supper), you will find options, but they are unlikely to be your favorite General Tso.

What about the salad bar's selections? Eggs? Eggs? I ate only the insides of the eggrolls and the crab rangoons. Unfortunately, those approaches leave a lot of wasted shells and deep-fried outside bits on your plate, and they appear to be a complete waste of food.

Wings anywhere—basic buffalo sauce, as well as Parmesan garlic, are usually fine.

Comfort stores are also a fantastic option! Hard-boiled eggs, cheese slabs, slim jims, almonds, and pork rinds are all available at 7-11. The pork rinds have a barbeque flavor and have zero carbohydrates.

Remember, whatever you desire, keep the potatoes, bread, noodles, rice, fries, and tortillas in mind. Additionally, keep an eye out for maize starch, bread crumbs, and other fillers. Balanced diet options and low-carbon alternatives are available, and a successful eating plan can be followed with careful preparation and excellent conduct.

For everyone, the ketogenic diet is a wonderful approach to lose weight. Visit Safe Keto, a helpful website that provides dietarians with meal ideas and dietary information.

CHAPTER THREE:

14. PLAN FOR A KETOGENIC DIET.

Ketogenic diets have exploded in popularity. It's an excellent approach to not only lose weight quickly but also to stay healthy and safe. For those who have tried and are now following the Keto Diet, it is more than just a diet. It's a new way of living, a whole different way of life. But, as with any major life change, it will take incredible dedication and determination.

For some, it's nice, but not for everyone?

—

While a ketogenic diet has been shown to dramatically improve quality of life, some people do not share the majority's viewpoints. But why is it the case? As we recall, the only method to lose weight was to avoid eating the unhealthy meals that we are accustomed to eating on a daily basis. So, if you tell individuals to eat healthy fats (the key word here is "healthy"), it's easy to see why they're unsure how and why they should eat more fat to lose weight rapidly. This concept contradicts everything we've ever learned about weight loss.

When it comes to modifying your diet, there's nothing to be afraid of if you're willing to embrace a little technology. For many people, changing their diet is a difficult task.

Particularly if they feel out of control, or if they are told they must follow a specific treatment to better cure a chronic ailment, or if they despise discomfort in the traditional sense.

The ketogenic diet is a popular weight-loss plan. It burns fat rather than glucose since it is high in fat and low in carbohydrates. The Atkins diet is well-known, but the ketogenic diet reduces carbohydrates even farther. Avoiding high-carbon foods can be difficult because we are surrounded by fast food and processed foods, but cautious preparation can assist. Here are a few of the keto diet's items.

15.Starting Points for You.

1.If you're only cooking for yourself, freeze or cool the remaining portions or, if necessary, split the recipes.

2. Feel free to swap lunch for dinner, breakfast for lunch, etc. on the same day. You can even switch the days completely if you want.

3.Make the keto buns ahead of time (the complete recipe of 10 can be made).

Freeze the night before or just before serving in the oven to keep it fresh. Defrost at room temperature.

4.There should be no need for snacks in between meals, but make sure you grab some keto-friendly snacks. Here's a list of snacks to try, as well as a whole diet list to round out your Keto Diet List.

5.Magnesium deficiency can occur on very low-carb diets (less than 30 grams of net carbs). I recommend taking magnesium supplements or eating magnesium-rich foods such as almonds. Also, take extra sodium (I use rosé Himalayan salt) if you have any keto-flu symptoms.

6.Minor adjustments to this eating plan are not required for everyone. If you need less protein, reduce the amount of meat and eggs you eat. Don't be concerned about a little more protein; you won't be kicked out. Protein satisfies hunger.

Concentrate on adding oils and fatty foods when adding more fat (or less) to your diet. Finding your ideal macros with KetoDiet Buddy!

7.Some recipes have higher total carbohydrates and fiber content. If you're concerned that fiber will sabotage your weight-loss efforts, consider the following: Total Carbohydrates vs. Net Carbohydrates: What difference does it make?

Fiber may assist you in losing weight.

8.If you aren't hungry, don't eat, even if it means you will have to store your food.

CONCLUSION

A good weight-loss diet is one that has no negative effects on your overall health. The truth is that some people prefer fad diets and end up jeopardizing their health. For example, while it is advisable to limit your carbohydrate intake in order to lose weight, completely eliminating the food group from your diet is not recommended. To match calories in and calories out, you must choose healthy carbs and consume them in the proper proportions.

Keto and low-carb dietitians understand the importance of planning ahead of time when visiting fast-food restaurants. It's nice to have some healthier options on hand before being tempted by menu items that aren't allowed on a low-carb diet. To make it simple to find a quick keto-friendly alternative, we've compiled a list of restaurants and fast food outlets, as well as items, that we've found to be the cheapest (and most emotionally satisfying) option. These aren't always the best options, but when you don't have any other options due to time or location constraints, they'll suffice.

To comprehend why the Keto Diet is harmful in the long run, you must first comprehend how the Ketogenic Diet works. A Keto diet is one that is very low in carbohydrates, which are one of the body's most important sources of nutrition.

www.ingramcontent.com/pod-product-compliance
Ingram Content Group UK Ltd.
Pitfield, Milton Keynes, MK11 3LW, UK
UKHW022011190726
13853UKWH00004B/1875

9 798423 212742